SIMILIA SIMILIBUS CURENTER

This is a light-hearted book about some of the situations into which a Homeopathist can be drawn simply by nature of the calling.

*It contains no case histories of registered patients, and as some of the contingencies dealt with have been 'on the fly,' or 'Good Samaritaned' detailed notes are not available, so 'The Bologna Express' should **not** be considered a text book or primer on 'best practice.'*

It does, however, show that Homeopathy can be used in crisis situations and in keeping with the light hearted nature of the book, a list of remedies used is provided at the conclusion of the book, but scrambled so that the serious student may draw his/her conclusions independently, if interested.

'The Tuscany Express' is dedicated to the great

Hahnemannians past and present - gratitude to Dr.

Margaret Tyler, Dr. Marjorie Blackie, Homeopathists,

and to my dedicated friends in orthodoxy, John

Vecchione, MD, Paul Jendrick, MD, and above all, to

young Niccolo who knows that HOMEOPATHY WORKS!

Contents

THE TUSCANY EXPRESS

I was on the Express from Firenze (Florence) to Bologna, travelling through the amazing Tuscan landscape, returning to my wonderful Star Vespucci Hotel outside Florence, when a young man walked rapidly down the corridor, looking into all the compartments and calling for a 'doctor.'

I introduced myself as a Homeopathist and offered my help should an orthodox physician not be available. As a guest in Italy I did not want to cause any offense to local medics nor injury to the good name of Homeopathy.

The young man said, 'please,' and guided me to a carriage a few 'doors' back, where a man in his late forties was huddled in fetal position on the seat, groaning with pain.

There were a number of people outside, and a couple of relatives inside. The young man introduced himself as a paramedic. I'll call him 'Angelo.'

He suspected the gentleman was experiencing a cardiac episode or arrest.

I asked for all but one relative to wait outside, and for a window to be opened and to loosen his clothing. His face was 'puffy,' feet and abdomen swollen, eyes yellow, somewhat bloodshot and bleary. I then took his pulses – as in 'Oriental' pulses, found anomalies on the Cardiac pulse; it was weak, intermittent and 'thready.' However his liver pulse was pounding.

During this time I asked questions, learned that he and his friends were partying all night in Florence, and were returning home.

For that and other indications, I provided one dose of the *indicated remedy*, waited to see if the 'picture' would clear or improve, and within *minutes* he was sitting up and ready to continue his journey.

His friends all crowded to the door, and cheered - most know about Homeopathy, and were vocal in their support! I had many invitations for libations from the generous Italians, but declined for reasons of protocol. I might accept those invitations today, however!!!

The Paramedic, Angelo, had judiciously called ahead to the nearest hospital, and after some wrangling, Sg Fiesta (Mr. 'Party man') very reluctantly agreed to break his journey and go to hospital for tests.

The train made an unscheduled stop. The ambulance was waiting at the station while a team of paramedics were waiting *on the platform with a gurney, or wheeled stretcher.*

An hour or so later, the Paramedic returned to my carriage to advise me that the hospital had contacted him to confirm that Sg Fiesta did indeed suffer cardiac arrest.

And people say that Italians are 'inefficient!'

THE MUSICIAN AND THE PLATE OF CALAMARI

If only they had told me about the fried Calamari!

It would not have changed the remedy.

It would have saved a visit to the Emergency Room.

A friend called to say his son was in distress. I don't usually respond to calls from persons not registered as patients, but I knew the family quite well.

It was a similar scenario to Sg Fiesta. Patient lying on the couch, groaning with pain, posterior left from lower angle of his shoulder blade to just above his waist line.

I saw his grandmother with acute cholecystitis (gall bladder attack) just as the medics arrived to take her for emergency surgery. I am certain that surgery was avoidable but my Homeopathic services were not required – just my 'comforting' presence…but that's another story. The poor woman was relentlessly cold, shaking under heavy blankets.

Back to hard working, much travelled Mr. RockBand!

I immediately thought of Nux Vomica, but did a quick anamnesis to see if another remedy 'peered through' the symptoms. The Pulse Diagnoses and concomitant symptoms confirmed a 'full ropey pulse' on the Gall Bladder meridian.

Indicated remedy - one dose only.

I was certain that Mr. RB avoided the alcohol and drugs associated with the entertainment industry and was otherwise healthy, so was puzzled by the severity of the attack.

Patient responded very quickly, so I returned to my apartment.

At 7 am the following morning I received another call.

Mr. RB had another attack, had spent the night in the ER of New York Hospital but they could not determine whether the pain originated in his kidney or gall bladder so they sent him home.

I dressed quickly and returned to their apartment. Mr. RB's pain had subsided somewhat but was still intrusive.

Suddenly I spotted a dish on the coffee table – a *giant dish of deep fried calamari!!!*

And yes, he'd scarfed down a plate-load before my first visit and was *feeling so much better after the Indicated Remedy that he started on a second portion...hence the second episode. This quickly and finally resolved to a second dose of the same remedy.*

Now the following always puzzles me:When a Homeopathist performs spectacularly or well, it's taken for granted but outside our beloved registered patients we are seldom given second chances.

For instance, the young man sat in the ER for hours *in pain,* while an army of highly paid staff took bloods, made X rays, poked, prodded, etc., and ultimately did nothing. Cost to insurance companies = thousands of dollars. Result = Zilch, Nothing, Nada!

Homeopathy initially cured the man within minutes, but I was not called in when his symptoms returned. Nor was an honest answer given when I asked if he had 'eaten anything unusual' that night.

If we start charging thousands of dollars for a visit – which Homeopathy is actually worth - we might engender more respect. On the other hand, we would miss so many wonderful patients and friends.

And I did 'break the rules, re treating persons who were not committed to Homeopathy - so I can't really complain when the wisdom of the historic Homeopathists triumphs!

SUFFERING IRISH...

My late husband, actor producer Dermot McNamara,

was invited to visit Tom and Pat King's house in

Connecticut.

It wasn't their property but a house that Tom was living

in while reconstructing it. Unknown to us, but in

retrospect not too surprising, was the fact that it was a

stealth base for extreme Irish nationalists. We were

lured there for the purposes of providing, for neither

money nor respect, our expertise to a bunch of yobos

who had stolen Dermot's theatre with the help and

support of City Council President Paul O'Dwyer, and who were also very well funded.

We were surprised to be picked up by a man under sentence of execution by the Official IRA for stealing millions from Bernadette Devlin's campaign funds, and shown to the back of a converted Post Office van. After a long, harrowing journey during which my imagination ran wild, we eventually pulled up outside a very nice Connecticut House complete with stables and paddock, unfolded our stiff limbs and breathed what was now the fresh, night air.

Pat, an ex nun, and Tom, a red headed 'viking,' gave us a snack and showed us to a nice room where we fell into a welcome, deep and profound sleep...

...shattered at an unearthly hour by the sound of a bodhran* outside our window and the chant: 'Suffering Irish, suffering Irish, suffering Irish Cath-o-lic!'

The tone of that chant made it very clear that the IRA were not invested in 'defending' or 'protecting' Catholicism in Northern Ireland.

They told us they were raising money for the 'Green Cross,' and were doing a street pageant based on Celtic legend at Lincoln Center.

A friend of Dermot's, a former owner of the Irish Pavilion, and sympathetic to the Provisional IRA later hissed 'I don't care what they tell you about band-aids and blankets – it's going for fookin' guns!'

And yet they received public grants denied to the Irish Players.

The 'pageant' gave them the 'background' to steal Dermot's theatre right from under his nose.

Suffering Irish indeed!

The rest of that story belongs elsewhere, but the memory of that chant echoed in my mind when I entered the refectory or dining room of a community of recovering drug addicts from around the world. Posted on the wall was a sign with the words: 'SUFFER SWALLOW SILENCE' or 'SWALLOW, SUFFER, SILENCE.'

They might as well have put 'Lasciate Ogni Speranza voi ch'entrate!'*

The addicts, many of them ill and infected with Hepatitis A, B, C slept in bunk beds, four to a small room. Bathrooms were limited and they were obligated to eat everything placed on their plate regardless of size or quality.

Since much of the food was experimental – eg, they were learning to make cheese from the milk of their donated cow – which some-how fermented, but was still forced upon them, the consequences were sometimes dire and the bathrooms in full use. Given that they lived 'on providence,' ie, donations, and were not permitted to ask for staples such as bathroom tissue, paper towels, etc., they were assured of considerable further suffering.

Only 15% were Irish, despite the majority of donations coming from Irish philanthropists.

***

They were caught between two stools: they were a community that lived a monastic, highly structured and penitential lifestyle, but they were *not* a religious community.

They were a group of recovering drug addicts under strict controls from their founder, Mother Elvira, but *under no local or national regulation.*

They were obliged to live 'on Providence' – while handsome donations went to the motherhouse.

Persons wanting to be formally involved, e.g., donate large sums of money, were obliged to go to said mother house, where, regardless of age or infirmity expected to participate in the life of the house.

Scrubbing floors until she was hospitalised did not appear to soften the heart of one elderly 'philanthropist' who did her best to alienate all other supporters irrespective of the consequences to the challenged addicts in recovery.

In this she was aided and abetted by the local GPs who told my patients that their complete cure of Hepatitis C was a 'Knock Miracle.' His associates, fans and admirers started a smear campaign against Homeopathy, to the effect that it was witchcraft, and not compatible with Catholic teaching.

Good thing they didn't mention that to Blessed Mother Teresa of Kholkata/Calcutta!

The young men of the community walked miles back from the local GP's office to my home to tell me that they was no trace of Hepatitis C in their systems, that the local GP said it was a miracle, but that they knew it was my work.

There is no Knock Shrine in New York and yet the same results prevailed there too.

*However, I believe that all healing comes from the Creator, and the system of Homeopathy while precise, methodical, and belonging to the highest order of Science, is **miraculous in its efficacy**.*

I wonder if the laboratory proof of my work at Knock is registered in the Vatican as a bona fide 'miracle,' because, by a strange 'coincidence,' my New York patients enjoyed the same success.

Knock Shrine pays said doctor E50,000 per year to verify miracles.

Further comment reserved.

PERSONA NON GRATA – for saving a young man's sight!

The leader of the rehab community was a Croatian, as

was his alleged second in command. This was,

however, a lie. The second in command was not the

other Croatian, but they broke all the rules, coming to

my house at 11 pm after a member of the community

was taken to hospital – allegedly – looking for espresso

coffee – and pain killers.

I told him Homeopathy didn't work that way.

We do not mask or block symptoms. We prescribe according to the *totality of symptoms* and treat the **root cause** of the problem.

Once that is resolved, the associated pain 'melts away.'

I was also acutely aware that they were addicts *in recovery* – without benefit of AA, NA, etc., programs which I highly recommend and concerned that they were off the wagon and looking for drugs. Their frequent visits to the DVD Rental store for violent movies, proscribed by the Founders of the community was one cause for concern. Adrenal stimulants lead to anxiety lead to temptation to re-use, a perilous situation for them.

They were not pleased that I had no analgesics and I started to wonder how serious this particular group were about their recovery.

Their testimony was pretty much the same – 'I hurt my parents, I'm sorry…' Whereas the testimony in AA and NA is deep, soul searching and diverse.

One system could certainly complement the other, but for some reason, Twelve Step programs were not allowed.

On a subsequent visit to their community, a young man, 'Ryan,' approached and asked to speak with me. He explained that was having problems with his eyes, and when he described his symptoms I told him he needed immediate treatment, and I would arrange a consultation with an ophthalmologist whose skills I was assured of, or would treat him homeopathically if he preferred. He chose the orthodox option.

Medical standards vary widely in Ireland without any real controls. Even litigation is prohibitively expensive. An egocentric physician would be quite capable of dismissing the concerns of a Homeopathist in order to protect his own reputation or downright prejudice, so I felt it important to bring him to a woman that I trusted 100%, and who was kindly but lived in Clonmel some one hundred and fifty miles away.

I told Ryan that I would make arrangements for him to see the ophthalmologist, should he so wish, and that I was willing to pay for his treatment.

Ryan thanked me, and the gentle Tipperary Opthalmologist said that of course she would see him. A priest missionary friend generously agreed to drive him.

And then all hell broke loose.

The Croatian lads said that Ryan could not see the ophthalmologist because the other rehab 'houses' didn't have a Homeopathist.

I asked if they were prepared to take responsibility for Ryan's complete and permanent loss of vision.

They still insisted that he could not see the ophthalmologist. There was some mention of the local GP, who habitually scoffs at my opinions, despite clear and unequivocal lab proof of Homeopathy's effectiveness, and who had apparently missed imminent danger to the young man's sight during his perfunctory *pro forma* screening of each candidate.

By God's grace there was a Youth 2000 conference in progress at the time, and the Spiritual Director of the Rehab House had returned from Peru for it.

I approached him and asked why they were willing to allow a young man, 24 years young, to permanently lose his eyesight.

Fr. Adrian was shocked and told me to tell them that Ryan was to see any physician that I chose and as soon as possible.

Ryan drove down a few days later with my dear Missionary friend, Fr. Martin, a Kiltegan priest, to Dr. 'Bernie' in Clonmel, where my suspicions of glaucoma were confirmed and his eyesight was saved. My friend in Clonmel, who refuses to be named, (but I've left a clue!) provided a prescription and report to the territorial local GP, and declined any payment for her service to the young man.

Due to the territorial 'sensitivities' of physicians in Ireland, Ryan's case was returned to the care of the local GP who continued to write the prescriptions recommended by Dr. Bernie and the young man's sight was saved.

I became suddenly *persona non grata* at the Rehab Community, and 12 out 15 members left in disgust, never to return.

I suspect that other abuses were going on, and wrote to the Religious Founders of the Community, who control from a distance but take no responsibility, despite demanding a high level of personal responsibility from their 'guests.'

Consequently, a system has evolved whereby letters to the Founders are intercepted and house leaders warned in advance.

The Founders may say that they 'didn't know' what was going on, and legally the young men are responsible for their 'houses.' However, the Founders decide who will be in charge, who gets moved around, and when and then step back to count the checks – or so it would seem.

The majority of the addicts in recovery are honourable; and subsequent leaders apologised to me, but the chinks in the armor need mending.

I have had the privilege of working alongside as well as for, some of the top specialists in the United States. Mostly American born and raised, these men put their patients' welfare ahead of bigotry and ego.

If the others realised how many malpractice suits we could prevent, the attitude to Homeopathy would change.

As is, however, authentic 'vocational' physicians do not have a problem with us; the battle is with Big Pharma who see profits plummet when patients are cured, whether by Homeopathy or 'unassisted miracles.'

To me, the system, inspiration and derivation of Homeopathy is nothing short of miraculous.

From the discovery of Cinchona (quinine) Bark by the Catholic Saint and Dominican friar, St. Martin de Porres of Peru, who named it for the Countess of Cinchon, a generous patron of his beloved poor, and sent it to

Europe via the Society of Jesus, or Jesuits, to the 'Eureka' moment of the great Samuel Hahnemann who saw that in small quantities *it cured the same symptoms that it created in large quantities or 'material doses!'*

With 'ruthless' Teutonic thoroughness, Dr. Hahnemann embarked on a scientific journey of discovery which generated an *explosion* of imitative and inspired research and innovation, much of which is ongoing today as many of his insights and findings are pirated and plundered and which gave us the profound and meticulous Science of Homeopathy.

Sci-tech is still catching up with what Hahnemann called 'The Gift of our Gracious God.'

Nothing 'New Age-y' there, my friends!

Would that orthodoxy had such Faith and Fidelity – we could work collegially for the betterment of humanity.

However, it is axiomatic that the more incompetent the physician – and there are some doozies out there – the more they will detest, despise and obstruct the work of the Homeopathist.

I fell foul of Dr. Nemesis, the Irish GP again, when I encountered a young man suffering a seizure on the floor of the Church.

The sacristan did not know what to do, and I did not have remedies on hand, but stood by to ensure that he did not injure himself.

In respect to the local 'territories,' and also because I believed the young man needed a CT or PET scan, I agreed that the worried sacristan should call the GP.

And so arrived Dr. Nemesis.

Angry at being called out – although it was his job for which, unlike me, he was well rewarded – he declared that the young man was drunk and that the Sacristan should call the police.

Now the young man had done no harm, had sought refuge and, apparently, healing, in the Church, and while the seizure had passed by the time Dr. Nemesis had arrived, the young man was still in a distressed state.

The police, aka, Gardai arrived, said 'ah, yes, this man is 'known' to us,' (a sure sign of guilt by Irish standards) and proceeded to pile him into their squad car.

I remonstrated, saying that he needed at least a EEC scan, but the Gardai rolled their eyes at Dr. Nemesis and said 'he's drunk!'

Even if that were so, alcohol toxicity can induce seizures and a tox screen should have been required before they dumped him in jail overnight.

I can attest to almost a dozen serious 'near misses' and misogynist abuse by said Dr. Nemesis who is paid by the local Church to prove and promote miracles.

In the meantime, he missed one rather spectacular one!

During the time that I spent in that area, the local Human Life International spent $16,000.00 to import a woman from the US, with no medical credentials whatsoever, to lecture and discredit all alternative medical systems competing with Big Pharma.

I could not fight this alongside superstition, venality, and such, limited my practice to known patients in the USA, and returned to writing.

I do, however, wonder how many lives would have been saved, had Dr, Nemesis had the integrity to send the lab reports to the appropriate Health Authorities in Ireland, and found one person with the courage to look further.

BROADWAY BLUES –HOMEOPATHY'S HEARTBREAK

The concierge of one of NY's finest and most celebrated hotels called me one night and asked if I would consult with a guest. This is one of the hotels in NY where one can frequently spot Secret Service men outside in all weathers, risking their lives for a WH official or foreign dignitary.

I was relieved to find that the call was not on behalf of a UN delegate from a terrorist sponsoring nation but for a well -known Broadway Actress rehearsing for an opening. We shall refer to her as 'BA.' Interpret

anyway you like.

It quickly became clear that not only was 'BA'

somewhat inebriated, but that she was not interested in

a consultation, but a drunken therapy session by phone,

no charge.

She was very agitated, anxious and upset, and knowing

actors, I tried to calm her without getting into details

about her relationship with her mom, or the day her

plant died.

Not trivialising any occurrence in anyone's life – for

example, the death of a neglected plant on the day that

a beloved teacher or neglected grandparent dies can

indeed trigger profound, reflexive issues of 'shame and

blame,' but Miss BA was not interested in resolving her

problems, only in dumping them.

I told her my fee for a house call – which was less than

one night at her 'hostelry,' and given the late hour in

NYC, more than reasonable – but she was not interested in providing professional respect or compensation, instead seemed to want a free therapy session on the phone which was not appropriate with a person whom I had never met, so I politely wished her well – as I do now – and hung up.

I was, however, sad to see that she was fired from the show the following week.

Penny wise – pound foolish!

TREATING THE ENEMY – a U boat Commander!

The daughter of a former U boat Commander, a German lady, 'Kay,' whom I greatly like and respect , asked me if I could 'do anything' for her father.

She told me, rather apologetically, that he used to lay mines along the English Channel, but quickly added that after the war he helped the British identify and remove them, and like many bona fide German military, detested Hitler and the Nazis.

Not enough to join the German Resistance – but then, already enlisted men hadn't a hope in hell of being demobbed.

Some time later she described the trek either near the end of WWII or just after, when they left their home near the seaport in Hamburg and took the long trail south to Berlin, for food. She spoke of the kindness of the British and the Americans to the German women and children, something she would never forget, she said.

Back to the patient – 'Vater' was diagnosed with Parkinsons, detested the medication and seemed to be having abreactions and becoming rapidly worse.

I asked a few questions about 'Vater,' diagnosed accordingly and two months later, Kay told me that 'Vater' no longer had Parkinsons, that the doctors believed they had misdiagnosed him, as he was walking about without tremor, rigidity, sign or symptom.

Thank God for Homeopathy!

ANTHRAX AND THE AFRICAN DRUMMERS

Back in the mid noughties there was a small, contained

outbreak of anthrax in NYC. It wasn't military grade and

the victims were unlikely targets of then 'careful'

jihadist groups, just students of African drumming, but

it was a scare and a puzzle.

NYPD 'tecs went to work and found a lone teacher of African drumming and importer of *skins* which he processed himself in his Brooklyn loft.

A former neighbour, whose children attended his class, discovered that her children were experiencing respiratory distress, packed them off the hospital where they were diagnosed and treated.

One did not suffer from the respiratory systems but had a nasty looking 'eschar' - a black scar- by her ankle, which persisted for days.

She turned to me for help. I made an exception to my 'registered patients only' rule as she was a fellow health professional asking for help for her child in distress, and so I treated the little girl.

The next day the eschar had disappeared and all but a faint pink tinge remained to tell of its existence.

I just wish I had taken before and after photographs.

Homeopathy can still surprise me with its rapid efficacy.

One of the children, a teenager, suffered from Sickle Cell Anemia. One of the concomitants of the illness is periodic retinal haemorrhage, impairing vision and putting the victim at risk of permanent sight loss.

'Could I do anything?' asked her mother.

One dose of the appropriate remedy and the following day and her vision was fully restored.

CHANNUKAH STORY – Torment and Triumph

One December morning, I received a call from a gentleman with a strong foreign accent. He wanted to make an appointment for his son.

His son was 42, he said and explained that his son was schizophrenic and that he would accompany him to my office, but remain outside in the waiting room during the interview.

His son was 'not dangerous,' he hastened to assure me.

*In my experience 'schizophrenia' is an amorphous, ill-defined mental anomaly, used as a brick with which to bash political enemies, independent minded intellectuals, malnourished genius, wounded survivors of child sexual abuse, addicts riddled by STDs and other infections, Irish Catholics (yes, Honey, they **are** talking about you – let's find a way to deal with it) and assorted other persons not willing to fit into pre-scribed boxes.*

It was the last appointment of the day and he was late, but just as I started to prepare to leave, there was a gentle knock at the door.

I said 'Come in,' and went to open it just as an elderly man peeked in.

He seemed distressed so I offered him a cup of tea and invited him to sit down, an invitation which he accepted.

He apologised profusely for his son's absence, said that his son was schizophrenic and difficult. He identified himself as a Holocaust survivor.

I told him that at Yad Vashem I learned that the children of Holocaust survivors had greater difficulty dealing with their parents' suffering than the survivors themselves.

It surprised and puzzled researchers and psychologists, or so our guide had stated.

He was surprised that I had been to Yad Vashem.

I'll call my guest Yacov, after an uncle in law who is named on Schindler's List.

There was a long pause, one of many during that afternoon. Then Yacov started to speak of his childhood in Poland.

He spoke of his mother and father, of his sister and brother, none of whom survived.

'We were happy,' he said, describing the lighting of the Shabbas candles, the friends who would come around and pray, the bright oil lamps, the food, the *abundance* of food, the prayers, the laughter, the music, the sharing...

He spoke about Channukah, the nine days of gifts, of celebration, of visits and visitors, of the special foods and their historic and sacred symbolism.

I do not recall their occupations, but the impression of his parents was one of educated, cultured people.

And the day the Nazis came and dragged them off.

He described the horror, the filth, stench, hunger, cruelty, sadism, abuse.

More pauses.

The death of his mother.

The murder of his father.

Silence.

We sat there, two strangers, tears rolling down our cheeks , in silence.

The horror and the sorrow were overwhelming.

It seemed as if a minute and an hour elapsed before Yacov could speak again.

This time he spoke of escape.

How he and some other small boys managed to elude the guards during the processing of new prisoners, slip out and run for it.

He was all of seven years young at the time.

The Polish Resistance helped them, and by various means of transportation, they found themselves on a train to Switzerland.

He said that when they saw Italian soldiers they ducked under the seats, and that there was some difficulty at the Swiss border, but they were eventually admitted.

Here there is a 'concurrence.' Iwo Herzer's moving 'The

Italian Refuge' describes an account by another refugee,

of Jewish children spotting Italian soldiers running

toward them and hiding under the seats as they halted

at a station near the Italian-Swiss border.

The soldiers were throwing hard objects at them, but

they were too frightened to look until the train started

up again.

Imagine the surprise of those poor children when they

saw that the 'missiles' thrown at them were actually –

candy!!! Sweets! Caramelli! They had not seen sweets

in years!

Ah, yes, 'the humanity of the Italians' of which Hitler

complained in an irate telegram to General von

Weisenheimer, his man in Rome. He was referring to

Mussolini's covert sabotage of all attempts to deport

Italian Jews.

I did not bring that up to Yacov. If he was one of those children, he was entitled to his memories, and if not, it would be too sad, another exclusion, another disappointment.

After the war he discovered that his siblings did not survive.

I left the questions aside, the 'research' questions – orphanage or foster care or kibbutz, or whatever.

They were, at that time, extraneous to occasion.

I just waited.

Yacov finished his tea, stood up and thanked me.

Tears were still rolling.

He asked what my fee was.

I said, 'no fee.'

He was surprised so when he offered again, I shook my head vehemently.

He shook my hand and said, 'thank you.'

I smiled and said,

'Shalom.'

He smiled, sunshine after the rain.

'Shalom,' he said, and left.

I never saw him again, but I hope he experienced some peace and love.

For myself, I received a possible answer to the question at Yad Vashem where they said

those who suffered intense bereavement and physical brutlity at the hands of Hitler's cohorts, were better adjusted than their children?

I conjecture that they had *safe memories.* They had the experience, vital to a child's sense of safety and inviolability, of 'parental omnipotence.'

They also had a safe and happy world to 'return to,' at least mentally.

That world, as hard as they try to pass it onto their children, will require generations to repair, to *feel* 'safe' again.

I do believe Homeopathy would have helped both him and his son, if allowed, but for Yacov, the most necessary 'remedy' was Love.

THE TINY, GREAT, BLESSED TERESA of CALCUTTA

There was considerable flak about Homeopathy which was gaining in strength in the USA in the eighties after a decade of one-on- one discussions with professionals in both the orthodox and alternative health fields.

The pharmaceutical industry with its 'dependency' medicine is a safe bet for investors – which is one powerful reason for the relentless assaults on the repeatedly proven effectiveness of Homeopathic Medicine.

Well, Big Pharma is a safe bet until one of the 'state of the art' 'double blind studies' is proven faulty and victims sue! Legal History and off-prime TV Advertising are full of such litigations.

'Double blind tests' are the stick used to abuse Homeopathy. However, 'double blinds' are inappropriate for such a refined, precise, patient specific protocol as ours. Besides, the protocols established by the great Dr. Samuel Hahnemann, and embellished and illuminated by his followers, have stood the test of two centuries now. The only product 'recalled,' ie, confined to 'prescription use only' is Arnica tincture – and whoever caused that recall is a greedy, child hating - fill in your own - expletive.

Ironically, the only people allowed to prescribe Arnica are the very persons completely ignorant as to its use, power and limitation, ie, the MD in thrall to Big Pharma.

That being said – we face another challenge with frauds and cheats. Just as Orthodoxy has its incompetents, we have to deal with **pseudo** Homeopathists 'reading symptoms off blue tubes;' prescribing on the basis of one symptom; prescribing multiple remedies – MD 'fashionable converts' are the worst for that – and so on.

However, sincere, patient committed MDs become outstanding Homeopathists.

In my files is a prescription made by a Park Avenue MD/pseudo-'Homeopathist.' She prescribed 15 *high potency* remedies, *per day*...for one patient.

I can only conjecture that she started to ab-use Homeopathic remedies in order to avoid killing off patients with Orthodox medicine and her incompetence.

She guaranteed, however, that some patients would never recover...even under the care of a *bona fide* Hahnemannian Homeopathist.

Which is why, when I encounter someone who says they 'tried Homeopathy and it didn't work,' I ask a few questions, and then can honestly tell him/her - 'you did not try **Homeopathy**.'

Radionics and Homeopathy

I'll give radionics its own paragraph, as my mentor, Lionel Roy Ogden of Cambridge, England, practised radionics and introduced me to Homeopathy. He did know his Materia Medica, and used a radionic block to facilitate the suffering people crowding his waiting room. I made an error by believing Carl Jung (I was 'jung' at the time) when he said that the picking of cards was not occultism but a resonance with the unconscious mind. (Memories, Reflections, Dreams) Of course when he wrote about entering his house and finding it choking with 'spirits' I should have run a mile.

Whether radionics is occultic, or whether a reflection of the unconscious, it bypasses the incredible teaching power of Homeopathy.   The search for the precise remedy and potency provides profound insight into the integrative nature of the human body; into the complexity of plant, animal and mineral life, and the complexity of its effect on the human body; into constitutional uniqueness; into heredity; the power of the body to repair itself and to the reality of our co-existence on this earth. Every organism, every mineral, every atom on this planet has been subjected to the same forces and stresses as the human person, and IMO, there is a unique *sympathy* between them and us, a *sympathy provided and used by our Gracious God to heal and strengthen us.*

Because of radionics, however, many Christians cast a dim eye on Homeopathy, believing it to be superstition, occultism and worse.

For this reason, I wrote to Mother Teresa, knowing that in India she would have encountered *bona fide* Homeopathists. In fact, an Indian Minister for Health, a Dr. Kumar, had invited me to India in the seventies.

About two months after I wrote this letter, there was a tap on the door of my office. I opened it and to my surprise and delight, two Missionaries of Charity were standing outside.

Naturally I invided them in – Sr. Sylvia and Sr. Priscilla, two of Mother Teresa's closest associates.

They invited me to assist their Missionary sisters in a Homeopathic capacity.

Naturally, I was delighted and found my life enriched and enhanced by the gentle Missionaries of Charity.

Some years later, as I was preparing to leave New York City, I emptied a book case and an envelope fell out.

It was addressed to Mother Teresa of Calcutta.

The letter had not been sent, and yet Blessed Mother Teresa of Calcutta had replied to it. St. 'Padre'

MEETING A SAINT

As I had consulted for the Missionaries of Charity, I was invited to meet Mother Teresa, now Blessed Teresa of Calcutta after a Mass for her sisters.

This was in Washington Heights, but I managed to find my way and work through the crowds surrounding the Church.

Because I was late, due to poor navigation on my part, I missed the group going directly to the Rectory via the Sacristy and had to go outside afterward, onto the street and back through more crowds into the Rectory.

The MC sister who opened the door, recognised me and squeezed me through a tiny aperture.

The late, great John Cardinal O'Connor was leaving as I entered and gave me one of his warm smiles.

I was then ushered into a small room along with M. Teresa's ophthalmologist – who had removed a cataract from one eye – and his family, and waited.

The late British journalist and convert, Malcolm Muggeridge, who introduced Blessed Teresa to the West, described filming her. His crew said that it was too dark, and the film would not 'take,' but that when she entered the room it was as if the lights went on.

When Mother Teresa entered the small ante room where I was waiting, the lights were already on – but when she walked in, *it was as if they had been turned up to a higher wattage!*

A tiny figure appeared accompanied by the late Sr. Sylvia entered and the room became suddenly brighter.

Sr. Sylvia introduced me and M. Teresa took my hand, placed a handful of Miraculous Medals into it and said 'Come and See me in Calcutta.'

She then placed her hand on my forehead. The rest deserves a chapter to itself.

When Mother Teresa touched my forehead, it was as if the floor, walls, and ceiling had melted away and I was 'standing' in the middle of eternity, in a dark but peaceful night.

I 'blinked' back to the present, but she had continued on to her ophthalmologist and his wife, also waiting for her. Sr Sylvia smiled over her shoulder. She was so warm and kindly. I did not realise that I would never see her again. She died in a car accident along with another of Mother's 'Saints,' Sister Kateri.

I waited for Mother Teresa to leave the room, made my farewells and left the building. As I exited the main door of the Church, I saw hundreds of religious and laity amassed outside and felt a strange sense of 'usurpation.' They were all so much more worthy of the meeting than I - until I realised that 'worthiness' had nothing to do with it. The reason became clearer a month later.

However on those steps I felt a strong surge of love for the people outside, and started to hand out the Miraculous Medals earmarked for friends and family posterity!

I had, for a number of reasons, developed a phobia about flying.

A few months after meeting Blessed Teresa, my brother invited me to his wedding in Spain. I reluctantly declined, but another family member insisted that I went, and bought tix on British Airways, knowing I trusted and once even enjoyed flying BA.

It was both a solace and exacerbation of my chronic homesickness for England. Yes, I know my fellow Homeopaths are 'screaming' the name of certain 'homesickness' remedies at me, and readers not raised in proto-terrorist 'cells' are –logically- thinking 'why not just go back,' but that's for another book.

At that time, too, Homeopathic remedies were not so easily available in New York City.

Well, the flight was booked for Good Friday! Penitential enough for the day, I thought, all factors considered. British Airways were kind enough to give us an upgrade to Business, which has forever spoiled economy class for me.

It being Good Friday, I requested a fish or vegetarian meal for myself, but on boarding was advised by Philip, named for one of Christ's Fishermen, that because of the special meal I could not avail of the upgrade.

The other family member said she would go back to economy as I was afraid of flying, and I said no, this was a big treat for her, and she said, well that was OK, so as we were debating who would enjoy Business Class on Good Friday, as other passengers struggled by, Philip rolled his eyes, went to the Purser and returned with assurances that we could both stay in Business Class and I would still get my piscine repast.

Later, as he served it, he advised me that they would bring me aloft to the cockpit after dinner.

Well it was a childhood dream to sit in the cockpit of a 747 in flight, but, but, but... I was now terrified at the mere idea, but still too committed to English 'good manners' to decline and follow my better instinct to hide under the seat!

After dinner when the lights were dimmed, Philip arrived with a lady crew member and a glass of champagne which they said to knock back, and they both directed me up the stairs and into the cockpit, where 'our chaps' - my childhood heroes, jolly English aviators, were cracking jokes about 'bumpy landings' and I literally felt like screaming and fainting at the same time.

Outside was just clear black starless sky, above, below, around, a cosmic emptiness interrupted only by the steady blinking of a line of lights crossing the Atlantic from New York to Europe.

I wanted to flee but was paralysed with fear. Bizarrely, the beauty of the scene was extraordinary.

Suddenly I was back in the room with Mother Teresa's hand on my head, and the sensation of the walls, floor and ceiling melting into eternity. A welcome peace came over me, even though physiological effects of 'jelly legs' remained, and I started to enjoy the silly jokes and the company of the successors of our great courageous RAF 'chaps.' We lost 14 every week during WWII.

Phillip returned to bring me back downstairs on my shaky 'pins' and the cabin suddenly looked like a large and comfy living room.

Later I had occasion to chat with Phillip in the galley.

When I told him that I believed my phobia was rooted in contact with some of my late father's associates, proto terrorists training in the Middle East, he continued food preparation for a moment, then suddenly froze for a moment.

He then asked me to repeat what I had said and when I did so, he told me he was a Protestant from Northern Ireland. *Like many Protestants and Catholics in Northern Ireland he had lost friends in the extreme violence perpetrated by the Provisional, pseudo, IRA.*

We shook hands and remained friends for the rest of the flight.

That was the day of the Good Friday Agreement when the IRA agreed to lay down their arms – in return for money, rights and privileges.

'Casualties' of the conflict, such as myself, with my invisible wounds, and, indirectly, Philip and others North and South of the border, were tossed aside for political expedience.

But I have flown thousands and thousands of miles since then with minimal apprehension. *Thank you, Mother Teresa!*

MOTHER TERESA and the ENGLISH PRINCESS

I had the opportunity to meet the late, sweet, Princess Diana, and did not 'seize it with both hands.'

Had I known that the following week her dying words, 'my boys, my boys,' would be splashed on headlines around the world I might have taken the opportunity.

The dear Sisters, Missionaries of Charity shared her last visit with me. They said 'Princess Diana was *like a daughter* to Mother Teresa.'

Their chapel is bare, spotless and beautiful. There is a large crucifix with the words 'I Thirst' above the image of Jesus, and a statue of the Virgin Mary. There are a few chairs for visitors or the disabled and elderly sisters.

The sisters sit on the floor during Mass and prayers. Many of their hymns are original both in music composition and in lyrics. When they sing, they sound angelic – as one would imagine a chorus of angels to sound.

When Princess Diana arrived, the sisters brought her into the chapel to wait for Mother Teresa. They brought a chair for her, placed it in the center of the chapel floor and sat around her, singing.

When Mother Teresa came downstairs, the sisters left, and they spoke for almost two hours.

Princess Diana was 'radiant' when she left Mother Teresa. After her death, a cartoonist depicted them walking up to Heaven hand in hand.

It was a sweet and consoling image for two sweet and consoling women.

ISRAEL – STILL THE LAND OF MIRACLES

My work brought me into contact with persons with disabilities, some still active in the work force, some, volunteering; others just getting by.

It helped me understand the difficulties of manoeuvring a wheel chair through NYC, getting up and down subway steps on crutches and wheeling rubber tires across acres of carpet in well- meaning but ill-advised hotels.

It led me to write about this in various news outlets for the disabled, and subsequently to Israel.

As a result of the many wars and acts of terror waged against Israelis in the last sixty plus years, Israel has a significant population of disabled soldiers and citizens. Added to the exigency is the antiquity of the cobbled streets, and the hilly slopes of some cities, e.g., Jerusalem.

However, every consideration has been made for chair users; while we were in the throes of the ADA act, Israel already had basic cuts and ramps at sidewalk crossings, etc.

Homeopathic remedies were available there too.

Which was just as well for a young, very attractive German TV journalist, 'Greta,' working for a French TV station and doing a story on Israel.

Our guide was a Berber, a former commando who guided the IDF members through the desert.

When I met Greta, her fair skin was red and blistered from the hot sun and desert treks. She was in considerable pain and discomfort.

Aloe used topically, brought her considerable relief, but it was the 'internal' Homeopathic potential (aka remedy) that astonished everyone.

The following morning, the blisters had disappeared, and her skin a pale pink, with minimal discomfort.

The Berber begged for the name of the remedy, but I did not tell him. I would prefer to give a course on Homeopathy than to provide the name of one remedy that might not be suitable for the next patient, and would then throw Homeopathy into disrepute.

On a different case, a different remedy might have been more appropriate. Homeopathy is too precise for 'one size fits all' prescriptions.

That being said, I used the same remedy for one of Mother Teresa's volunteers, a supermarket manager, who sustained a chemical burn to his eye from a splash of lye, and was in considerable pain and discomfort for a couple of days. The following morning he called to thank me and say that his pain was completely gone and his vision was fine.

Small miracles in Israel – for example, the threat of rain almost forced the guide to cancel the trip on Lake Kenneret (Gallilee). I suggested we 'ask the Prophet Elisha' to hold off the rain, and he did – until the guide started talking about Baptists jumping into the lake in the middle of thunderstorms. One of our group members said it would be exciting to see a storm and imagine Jesus walking on the water toward St. Peter, and suddenly lightning pierced the sky, and a storm broke.

It lasted a few minutes, but delighted the pilgrims and writers present!

Another 'small' miracle happened along the Via Dolorosa. I was making a photo record of the Stations of the Cross, most of which were marked. The Ninth Station however, where 'Jesus meets the Women of Jerusalem' took place where the cobbled roadway intersects with a market place and posted no signs.

"I'll photograph it anyway," I thought, raising my camera – *just as a flock of white veiled young women 'appeared from nowhere' and stood in front of it!*

As G.K. Chesterton once wrote: *'To those who have Faith, no explanation is necessary, but to those who have none, then no explanation is possible!'*

Again, in the desert on Mother's Day, sitting on a rock, feeling rather blue and guilty for not being with my teenagers – presumably piling up used dishes and pizza boxes pending my return – I was delighted when a partridge suddenly appeared out of nowhere, a mother hen followed by her five chicks. They walked toward me and I remained very still as they passed closely by me and disappeared again.

It was as if God patted me on the shoulder and said, 'it's OK, 'Mom,' you'll see your chicks again…'

I do not know who, in the Israeli Ministry of Tourism, or El Al, made the arrangement, but I am eternally grateful for the First Class upgrade on the return flight.

'Welcome Home' said the immigration officer at the JFK El Al Terminal as I bounced off the long flight, so tanned and fit that my neighbors didn't recognise me!

And yes, the pizza boxes were waiting…

'Welcome Home' indeed!

My visit to Israel has some bearing on the second visit
of the Holy Father, Pope John Paul II to New York City.

As guests of El Al Airlines and the Israeli Tourist Board, I
and a group of writers were invited to observe 'routine
maintenance' on one of their 747s.

Every three years, their jets are gutted and re-
assembled screw by screw, thread by thread, wire by
wire, every single item counted and accounted for.

One of the mechanical engineers was a Russian wearing
a Guinness t-shirt!

As I was invited by reason of my interest in and work
with persons with disabilities, the El Al execs took great
pride in showing me their 'ElAlift.' It was years back, so
I'm not sure if the spelling is correct. It's probably
standard now, but it was unusual then, a lift using a
'scissors' fulcrum to bring wheelchair users from the
ground to the boarding area.

Shortly after my return, I bumped into Cardinal O'Connor's Secretary, a gentle Monsignor with an eidetic memory and a huge heart who is now an Archbishop, an Archbishop who came from the pomp and circumstances of his Episcopal Ordination in Rome to a public hospital ward to administer last Sacraments to a prostitute dying of AIDs. Wow!

At the time of our encounter, everyone was asking for the return of John Paul II, so I took advantage of the meeting to ascertain if, and when, John Paul II might visit New York City again.

Monsignor shook his head sadly, and mentioned that since the attempt on John Paul's life, he was unable to climb the steps required to ascend to a platform where he would be visible to all.

"What about an El Alalift?" I asked, not ready to give up.

"El Alalift?" he asked quizzically.

I was sure he had places to go, people to see, but this kindly man never, ever, gave the impression that there was any other person in the world but the party that he was addressing.

I explained El Alalift to him, and he listened carefully.

I hope El Al doesn't mind too much, but I also suggested that they might lend him one.

He thanked me and went on his way.

A short while thereafter, it was GAME ON!

Announcements were made, and dates were set.

The Holy Father, John Paul II, was on his way!

Whether or not the El Alalift was used, it was inspirational!

Whether or not the confluence of circumstances was coincidental or a 'succession of small miracles' is debatable.

However, as GK Chesterton once wrote: *To those who have Faith no explanation is necessary, to those who have not, no explanation is possible!*

Or, as scripture puts it 'His eye is on the sparrow...'

This heroic man eventually became a registered patient, but I first encountered him in the Respiratory Unit of a municipal hospital in New York, visiting him at the request of the chaplain, the late, much missed Timothy Healy, SJ.

He was in agony; hemiplegic - one side paralysed after a stroke, fed by a stoma, or tube, surgically inserted into his stomach, attached to a respirator and subject to constant infection. Furthermore, he shared a room with at least three other patients, some of whom were more alert than he and had no compunction about turning the volume on their boom boxes (CD/radios) to intolerable levels.

He had endured this for eighteen months!

In addition to which, as I discovered later, one or two members of the nursing staff made his life miserable once they understood that he was a Catholic priest.

Had these racists understood that he was a Coptic Rite Bishop of Egyptian Birth and Turkish heritage, they may have restrained themselves.

An element of anti-white racism permeated the municipal hospitals that I knew well; the local politicians kept an eye on grass roots public jobs and stacked them accordingly.

I started to visit him regularly; at one point discovering him in a separate room stretched out as if on a cross, and surrounded by medical personnel –'centurions' trying to stick nails, ie, needles into his feet and hands in an effort to located an undamaged vein.

He had chronic infections, a result of the treatment rather than the illness, and, from observation, I was certain that I could help him.

After discussion with the Director of Respiratory Medicine, the Provincial of the Order, and his 'Next of Kin' who was also an MD, and the Archdiocese to whom he had been seconded, and of course, the Coptic Monsignor himself, it was agreed that I start treatment.

One week later he was free of infection. A month later, on room air, i.e, off respirator all day, until evening time.

Two months later he was wheeling himself about the hospital, concelebrating Mass and one month after that, he was down again.

His brother had persuaded him to undergo the implantation of a Diaphragmatic pacemaker, still in development/experimental stage, and so after two months of freedom, the dear man was under the knife. The rationale being that the Med Director was understandably cautious about the risk of sleep apnoea. Then again, despite his professional affirmation of my work, he didn't really know just how much a Hahnemannian Homeopathist can do for a multiply compromised patient.

I was certain that had he remained exclusively under Homeopathic treatment, that he would eventually have left the hospital and returned to his mother house, but I realised that the orthodox physicians were highly conscientious and did not know enough about Hahnemannian Homeopathy's spectacular results to trust us completely.

Despite the compelling evidence before their eyes. And so my unspoken fear that he would not return to active duty at his Provincial House was fulfilled.

With Homeopathy's help, however, he recovered quickly enough from the surgery, and without further infection or complication was moved from the Respirator Unit to the Nursing Home Unit at a saving to his Insurance provider of $1,000 **per day.**

Without Homeopathy, this would not have been possible.

While my dear friend did not permanently leave the hospital, he subsequently enjoyed many visits to his Provincial House, to his Coptic Church and to the Holy Father, John Paul II's Masses.

The Administration, once apprised that such an erudite gentleman was in their Nursing Home unit, provided him with a large single room overlooking the river, where he became a valued and beloved volunteer chaplain for his remaining years, on call 24/7 to staff, visitors and his fellow patients and residents.

Coincidentally he had attended seminary in Lyons, France, which has a world renowned Homeopathic Pharmacy. If his 'Cause' goes forward I'd like to 'claim' him as the Patron Saint of Homeopaths!

THE COPTIC MONSIGNOR AND THE HOLY FATHER

At the Aqueduct Raceway, five husky Franciscan friars carried Monsignor's wheelchair up five flights of steps to the platform where the priests would concelebrate the Sacred Mass with the Holy Father.

As we waited, a flock of doves rose and dived around a tree, moments before JPII's chopper arrived and landed on the ground outside the platform.

I stood up and looked over the side.

The Holy Father, John Paul II stepped out of the chopper and looked up directly at me.

I froze. There were no protocols for greeting a Pope at my childhood English private school.

'Should I curtsey?' I wondered, staring at the Holy Father.

His face broke into a megawatt smile, and he waved, and I waved and that smile is forever in my heart.

Central Park

I did not need the five husky friars to bring Monsignor to the Central Park Mass, but they were there, helpful as ever, and afterward we enjoyed the hospitality of none other than the Grand Duke of Austria and his beautiful, American wife, Elisabeth!

One of Geza von Hapsburg's forebears was the great saint, Princess Elizabeth of Hungary, whose services to the poor and Franciscan generosity and simplicity arelegend. He and his wife are gentle, kind, hospitable souls.

The young friars had spent the previous night sleeping on the floor of their Lexington Avenue apartment – large by New York standards, but not sufficient for half a monastery!

I suspect that they offered to host them in a hotel, but the friars, true to their Franciscan spirituality, would decline that.

The Mass itself was interesting – concelebrating priests sidelined then Police Commissioner, William Bratton, sidelined, and outside the 'celebrity zone,' while what seemed to be the brashest stars on Broadway challenged the goodwill of the devout congregation sitting on grass, or uncomfortable folding chairs while waiting for the real star, John Paul II.

The Holy Father finally arrived to outstanding applause and relief!

He must have read our hearts, because, during an address to us, he suddenly broke out into a beautiful Polish Christmas Carol, in a strong, unaccompanied, a capella voice.

After that, everyone settled and the Mass continued with due reverence.

When I returned him to the hospital, seven hours after 'springing' from his ward, the indomitable Monsignor, who had to rise at five am and miss at least one 'in stoma' feed of Ensure for at least four hours, thanked me profusely and then said wistfully,

'I so wish I could attend the Rosary!'

'No more tickets, no special passes,' I replied, sad to disappoint him, but glad to 'put my feet up,' so to speak.

He must have had a 'hotline to Heaven,' because when I returned to my apartment there was a Special Delivery package from the Archdiocese of New York with... passes to the Rosary!

Hmmm

And so we went, again, up at 5 am, one feed for the morning, over the river, across the sidewalks, along the avenues of New York and through the police barricades surrounding St. Patrick's Cathedral.

And the previous year he'd been stretched out on the hospital bed for eighteen months, unable to speak or move any part of his right side; now he was wheeling his chair independently, sipping beef broth and diluted orange juice, blessing his friends, hearing confessions, speaking through a trach tube, breathing normally – except when they put him on a precautionary respirator at night.

I was hoping that Monsignor would have the opportunity to meet John Paul II, and I am certain that had I been able to apprise the late, great hearted Cardinal John J O'Connor that the Coptic Monsignor would attend the Holy Father's rosary, then Cardinal O'Connor would have arranged for him to be at the Sanctuary with his brother priests.

It was not meant to be. Or perhaps some overwhelmed usher 'got in God's way,' but it was still a delightful, prayer-filled and profound experience.

The same lovely Englishwoman, Anne, at the Archdiocesan Office of Disabilities, who sent the 'Hail Mary' tickets, had also provided tickets for two of my dearest, disabled patients.

To their delight, the Holy Father stopped by their pew and took their hands.

He didn't have to know their story. He read their hearts. That is one of the hallmarks of sanctity.

The staff at Goldwater Hospital deserve a gold medal award for going off routine in order to facilitate Monsignors 5am preparation and 6 am departures.

They had some bad apples, certainly, but the majority were dedicated and compassionate. Shining stars in the firmament of hope.

At last report the hospital was undergoing conversion into luxury apartments overlooking the East River and facing the UN. Patients were shipped to the suburbs and upstate; for many of them losing their home of many years, their orientation and their mates.

THE CASE OF THE AIRSICK AIR CREW

Vincit Omnia Amor!

Love conquers all? Not in the case of the air hostess and her pilot boyfriend.

A low fare special to Italy. The 'sardine can' effect. Maximum income for minimum outlay. Hundreds of holiday makers jammed into a small jet with one narrow aisle. The inevitable hustle to sell drinks and food…

…along with apologies for the delay in service.

One of the crew members was air-sick in the back of the plane; another crew member was helping her. This always happened at the beginning of the flight, but she was usually better by the end…

And why did she continue to fly?

Her boyfriend was the pilot and this way they could 'layover' together.

Interesting choice of words, given that particular 'budget' airline offered very few 'layovers' to its crews.

Did I know anyway to help her?

Short of keeping her feet on the ground, er, yes.

'See a Homeopath.'

'Is that herbs and stuff?'

'No, that's Homeopathy and science.'

'Are you one?'

'Yes.'

'Can you give her something?'

'I don't even know her...'

'I'll see if she'll come up to you...'

'That's ok. Is she fair, skinny and...?' I asked, not wanting to 'lead' her.

'No, she's fair and, not exactly plump, but...'

'Sitting down and a glass of water – would that help?'

'No, it's when she sits down for take-off it starts and the water just sets her off...'

Anything else? Anything unusual?

More out of compassion for the crews that had to double up while working for a less than kindly boss, I wrote 'See a professional Homeopathist about this,' and the name of the remedy that I considered appropriate on a card and gave it to the concerned friend of the air-sick, love-lorn stewardess.

No feedback, no thanks expected.

On a number of occasions I have helped other passengers by using acupressure points to temporarily relieve anxiety, particularly with smokers undergoing withdrawal.

There are Homeopathic remedies, but without a commitment it is a waste of time and energy to treat the casual and uninformed, unless the situation is acute or critical.

Chamomile tea is helpful in such situations, but few airlines carry it, and few smokers of my acquaintance like it! A breakfast of oatmeal is also calming, and provides essential stamina to see passengers through today's stressful airports.

Persons with any form of anemia should board as late as is courteous and possible as 'clean air' standards have dropped considerably – offset on the other hand, by proscriptions on smoking.

Nothing works better and with a stronger opportunity for permanent recovery than Homeopathy, especially where the condition is Constitutional.

Another overseas excursion took me to Germany to a conference on Science, Religion and Philosophy.

We arrived at Munich Airport and were driven by luxury coach to a town in the foothills of the Bavarian Alps. It was stunningly beautiful, a cross between The Sound of Music and one of those scenes where allied soldiers come across a beautiful meadow, let down their guard until the greenswards turn red to the sound of machine gun fire.

The EU wants us not to 'mention the war,' but its shadow still looms over a coercively united Europe.

Walking into town, we suddenly found ourselves approaching rail tracks and stopped in unison, standing speechless for a moment, then exchanging glances in frozen silence, collectively remembering The War – the movies, the news reports, the broken relatives.

At the time, we were all strangers.

Another reference to the war occurred when older women would approach like Panzer tanks and try to push me off the road. It was so frequent that the gallant men in the company would start to block them.

After two days of this, once the jet lag wore off I realised that my tiny British-American flag pin was probably evoking very painful memories, and so, reluctantly, I removed it.

My English childhood was happy, so the flag pin represented good cheer.

However younger Germans feel about the war and its postlude, it was clear that the elderly were still in pain.

As a later visit to Dachau showed, it took twelve years of bullying, assault, kidnapping, murder, smashed presses, 'disappearing people, etc., by an Austrian usurper, to turn the people of Germany into compliant, robotic Nazis.

Was my flag pin insensitive, or was it a form of self defence? I took a stop-over in London so that I could arrive in Munich on British Airways.

The truce may be signed and the elites go out and celebrate, but the people of lesser privilege, who clean up, rebuild, tend to the injured -'get on with it,'so to speak - carry their wounds, visible and invisible, to the end of their lives.

And, as with the innocents of Auschwitz, pass them on to their children.

As we sat down for a supper of processed meats, cheese, bread and coffee a harried looking man joined us. He seemed intelligent and introduced himself as 'Ivan,' a paediatrician. He was not one of the Eastern Europeans at the conference, some of whom had different motivations for attending the conference.

As he did.

The following day, after a breakfast time imitation of the scatty White Rabbit in Alice in Wonderland, he confided to me that he had come to Germany to commit suicide.

Silence, any cynics out there! Even when hyper rational as in authentic OCD (Obsessive Compulsive Disorder) mental health issues are by definition, *irrational.*

Dr. Ivan spoke of his addiction to prescription drugs, supplied by his medical friends, and that he was 'on withdrawal' and would be happy to undergo Homeopathic treatment.

Oh yes? Oh no!

Talk about being between a rock and a hard place!

The 'enemy' had crossed camps and sought my help but at what a price!

Perhaps requesting my professional help was his insurance policy – to prevent me from going outside professional limits...to personally compromise me and my work.

He assured me that he had gone cold turkey, was undergoing withdrawal, and would accept my protocols. I took him at his word. I mean, who wouldn't trust a paediatrician.

At least till I observed him ogling the body of a child gymnast/circus entertainer clad only in a leotard performing aerial lifts, etc., with a much older man, on the chilly streets of the Czech Republic.

Still in Germany I was very frustrated with the progress of Dr. Ivan. His face would brighten and vitality return within a few minutes of the 'well chosen' remedy, but every morning he arrived at the breakfast table, addled, 'hung over,' confused, muttering to himself...

...still denying use of narcotics, psycho-tropes, etc.

Hmmm

He had played a strong sympathy card. With his 'suicidal intentions' hanging over me like a sword of Damocles, I was reluctant to abandon him. He had become dependent on our evening walks, even as the other 'devout Catholics' started to gossip about an 'affair,' and asking who was the woman leading this good 'married man' astray, etc.

'Ivan's' grandfather supported Hitler, he said. His first wife committed suicide, leaving him with 10 kids to raise; she was schizophrenic, he said. He re-married, an ambitious woman with two young daughters, one five, one eight, and a redneck ex-husband with whom she was still 'friendly.'

He started to extol the beauty of the little girls in their 'marching band' outfits and their 'gymnastic outfits.'

Later, in Prague, I was to wonder if the little gymnast reminded him of his step daughters or if something else was on his mind.

Something he had to shut-down with pills, perhaps.

In Prague the musicians, street, church, whatever and wherever, were outstanding. The mechanical clock was amazing. The restaurants were full of duck: duck a l'orange, duck aux cerises, duck - and duck and duck...

The rivers weren't.

The hotel menu's choice of vegetable was: carrot, carrot, or carrot.

'Thank you, I'll have the carrot!'

Prague to me will be the eternal cold and damp and cold. I'm sure that it has developed beautifully since that long ago visit, but the memory of standing in damp, run down churches and walking slowly through the town squares chills me to the bone to this day.

It was late Spring, and as I expected to be staying exclusively in Bavaria, which is Southern Germany, I brought only a light jacket. The chill had started when we crossed into former East Germany and across the still bleak landscape into the even more forlorn terrain of the new Czech Republic. The ice queen of Narnia must have represented *Communism, a brutal system that turned all to stone* and the 'statues' were only slowly returning to life.

Dr. Ivan expressed some concern for me, wrapped his jacket around me and offered to bring me back to the one star-no star hotel to which we had been assigned and which possessed an abundance of carrots.

The round-about journey was via a taxi driven at high speed by what appeared and sounded like a former KGB hitman, with an array of porn photos on his dashboard.

I had enough of his whirligig navigations and spoke sternly in Russian.

Dr. Ivan looked like he wanted to dive under the seat, but 'KGB' taxi-driver sat up straight and said 'Da,' and brought us quickly and directly to the hotel. The Iron curtain may have fallen, but the 'imprint' of the 'Iron Maidens' of the Soviet underbelly was still as chilling as the landscape.

At the hotel, Dr. Ivan went into over drive. He insisted on bringing warm drinks to my room, brought extra blankets, and decided he should stay to 'observe' in case I developed a fever. He sat in an armchair as I fell asleep feeling cared for.

'Ivan' fell asleep too, in his armchair until...

We awoke to a banging on the door.

Had KGB come to exact revenge?

"Don't open it!' said Dr. Ivan.

"Dr. Ivan! Dr. Deirdre! Are you in there!"

It was an American voice. One of our company. I was about to open the door, but 'Dr.Ivan' grabbed my arm.

"Don't open it!" he pleaded, "someone might tell my wife!"

"Tell your wife what?" I asked, puzzled at his newly manifest panic. The circumstances were innocent on my part at least.

"That I, that I..."

"That you fell asleep helping a friend - besides who here knows your wife?"

Most of the company, it turned out.

"But what if someone is sick and needs you or I? Besides, they will come to their own conclusions anyway with *both* of us unavailable..."

"I will say we went to a nightclub..."

"That's better?"

"You don't understand," he said.

"You're right," I thought, "I don't."

The following morning at the breakfast of carrots, er, rolls and coffee, carrots and more carrots, as I entered the carrot room from one direction, and he from another, seating himself at a different table, there were a few interested glances, brief and polite.

One of the group leaders came in, saw us, and came over to me. Mrs. 'Beauregard' was ill last night. We were looking for you.

'Mrs. B?'

A stout, reticent mature woman with dark brown hair, unhappy since her arrival in Germany. She –wisely- took to her room in Prague and was not visible during our walkabout the once glorious city.

"She had some, er, abdominal pain," he said, a good Catholic male highly uncomfortable with 'womens' issues,' - "if she doesn't recover we'll have to bring her to the Canadian Clinic, and stay in Prague for up to three more days…"

"The Canadian Clinic?" I asked to mask my rising panic at the prospect of three more days in the Carrot House Hotel. Did I mention the plumbing? Or the confabulated contraption masquerading as a shower?

"It's the only, er, Western style medical service in Prague. I don't know what you can do, but…"

"No you don't know what I can do," I thought.

"…but will you at least see her?"

"Of course – did you ask Dr. Ivan?"

"Yes."

"Of course, you asked him first…!"

"And?"

"He said he was a paediatrician."

"Interesting," I thought, as the organiser led me to Mrs. B's room and left me there.

She was still in agony – Colon pulse full and bursting, Small intestine pulse tense and wiry; excess yin, insufficient yang…

Mrs. B had been 'blocked' since arriving in Prague, and a few days prior. The bus journey was agony, every jolt painful; In bed, every movement was an effort, and aggravated her pain.

She was quietly assertive, a woman accustomed to her own way, but without being obnoxious. Later I learned that she was an heiress to a 'small' shipping fortune. There was none of the tentative reticence of the *Nat mur* 'tremblors' which would point to the hypernatremic (high sodium) diet of the Bavarian hostel – a four star hotel by contrast with the Carrot House – so I understood that something deeper was going on with Mrs. B.

After asking a few discreet questions, administering the appropriate remedy, and working on her meridians via acupressure, I tip toed out, allowing her to sleep.

The following day she was fully recovered and ready to travel at the scheduled time.

She thanked me and told me to bill her insurance company in New York.

Getting back to Germany was thanks enough.

The bus ride was 6 hours – long enough for me to notice a different kind of 'chill.'

The 'chill' of exclusion by the married women who assumed that the slender New York Homeopathist had seduced the poor innocent Dr. Ivan and 'had her way with him.'

They would make sure 'the trollop' didn't spend the night with *their* husbands!

With good reason! Some of the husbands – who had jumped to the same conclusions – were noticeably warmer after the week-end in Prague!!!

Perhaps in appreciation for their wives' renewed 'romantic interest!' Perhaps not!

I was educated in England where the Royal Motto is:

'Honi soit qui mal y pense!'

Shame on him who evil thinks…or as the Scriptures admonish: 'To the pure all things are pure!

Persons of Faith will appreciate the following anecdote: There was a hold up at the Czech-German border. The bus driver said it could take 8 hours to get through. There were 'industrial' public bathrooms at the border area, otherwise we would be stuck on the bus for eight hours – and at European petrol prices, the engine would not be idling.

Another chilly evening and six hour drive in the darkness for a total of 15 hours travel time.

The baby on the bus was crying and crying. Her parents could not get her formula opened, and the small gift kiosk at the border did not have the right opener. None of us had what was, essentially, a 'beer key.' No, they were not feeding beer to their baby! The packaging was unusual, perhaps Czech, perhaps German, probably not American.

The baby's cries melted everyone's hearts. I turned to my immediate neighbours on the bus and suggested that we pray the Rosary.

By the time we had reached the 5th decade (about 10 minutes) the bus driver announced that the blockade had cleared and the bus would be moving within 20 minutes.

He also made a stop on the German side where the parents of the hungry child acquired an opener.

Win win.

For the fearful flier – the rosary is also effective with turbulence. Pretty much anything benign, in fact!

I was invited to visit a hospital for alternative medicine in Munich. Dr. Ivan expressed a strong interest in accompanying me, so to the alarm of the group, we disappeared for the afternoon. More scandal!

Many German towns have a Bahnhopf and a Stadt by the same name, so if you don't know the system you can end up on the wrong express heading toward another region entirely.

We did make it safely to Munich, and while the Medical Director welcomed me cordially, I was disappointed to see that they were not doing the level of work that I had the privilege of attaining in New York.

Most of the patients whom we saw were suffering from joint disease and had worsened on orthodox medicine. They were mostly out patients.

I was hoping to see the dramatic and challenging cases that I had read about from the early days of Homeopathy, before Big Pharma spuriously closed down our hospitals and faculties.

Still it was good to see a hospital designated exclusively for Alternative Medicine.

At Munich the station was large and spotless. On acquiring tickets for our return, the attendant handed us a print out with the name of the train, the carriage numbers, the name, rank and serial number of the gentleman who had painted the train...er no! I exaggerate, but the shadow of the war and the efficiency of the rail network seemed inextricable.

What was totally unexpected was the good nature and good humor of the German train conductors and station masters, all of whom spoke excellent English, even those assigned to rural stations.

Our 'laddie' had a shaved head and ear-ring and looked rather menacing, but laughed his head off at the final stop when he learned we had missed our destination, now thirty miles behind us. We had taken the express rather than the local. One served the 'Stat' station and the other served the 'Bahnhopf,' but you'll have to call Munich to find out. I certainly can't tell you, but they will speak excellent English, and they will know exactly what track, number, carriage, etc., that you will need and which station is which.

They just won't know that you don't know that the ticket you are purchasing may be for the wrong train entirely!

The German for train is zug zug.

Cute.

THE PARANOID PEDIATRICIAN AND THE PILE OF PROZAC

My faith in Homeopathy is such that when I do not get the positive results expected from a careful prescription, I start to suspect 'interference' from orthodox sources.

'Ivan's' relapses were baffling.

He would be fine after the remedy to the end of day – until the following morning!

At the end of the seminar, the expected transformation from worried, paranoid, suicidal persona to energised, optimistic, life affirming professional had not taken place.

I learned that after our long sessions, he would sabotage the effects by engaging in long, transatlantic diatribes with his distant wife.

That was certainly his prerogative, but I started to wonder why he would claim that his marriage was over when it was still very much alive - rancorous, but dynamic, and abuse my therapeutic skills and time, if the relationship had not ended.

I wondered what else he was not truthful about.

He said he could not consult a psychiatrist or see a counsellor about his ideations because in his State, that would put him at risk of being struck off the register.

But his psych colleagues provided him with ample supplies of unsupervised psychotropes.

He claimed to have discarded all his medications, but his addled confusion, and periodic short term memory lapses suggested otherwise.

Still he insisted.

On the last day of the seminar, I went, for the first time, to his room, to return a book.

It was morning, before breakfast and I tapped on the door. Fortunately another member of the group was observing from her balcony. Otherwise anyone seeing me emerging from Dr. Ivan's room at that hour would assume the worst.

The taste for scandal in supposedly Christian communities is, in itself, scandalous!

The Dr. opened it, looking dishevelled, even addled.

He seemed frightened, checked the street, like a character in a B spy movie, and ushered me in.

"What if someone saw you coming in here!"

"Someone did!"

"Who? Who?"

I mentioned the lady on the balcony opposite and asked what was the problem.

Before he could answer, my gaze landed on the coffee table which was literally *covered with prescription psychotropes, including a pile of boxes of Prozac – with prescription labels, yet!*

"You should have told me," I said, "I would not have wasted my time and energies…"

"No," he insisted, "You helped me, you really helped me. I am going back to try and make my marriage work. My family depend on me."

I don't like failure. Even when it's not mine. He was still addicted. And Prozac was still complicit in the suicides of its users.

Homeopathists need to know *everything.*

Then again, he 'sobered' up long enough to rethink his marital status, and no longer saw suicide as the only way out.

The assembled company, each of whom was dealing with different issues, would not return to their desolate Eastern European enclaves, their industrial North American enclaves and their declining European Union satellites with the shadow of the doctor's suicide hanging over them.

Instead, they returned with what they believed to be a juicy scandal!

Oh well!

Whatever floats your boat, as my friend Lisa says!

OBSERVATION

Under the influence of Prozac and a 'moderate' amount of alcohol, a male acquaintance committed a reprehensible felony; under the influence of another psychotrope, another male acquaintance likewise committed a felony. A female Buspar and Beer abuser abducted a child.

These persons were all reputable persons of good standing in the Catholic Church.

A gentle Buddhist on Synthroid was exposed to marijuana smoke and went berserk.

From what I know of them, it seems that their medications and/or meds plus alcohol, played a significant role in their aberrant behaviour.

The abuse of psychotropes developed as 'chemical restraints' for persons incarcerated for mental illness must be re-evaluated in a civil world, but until we put people before profit, we cannot claim to be either civil or civilised.

'If it is from God it will endure…'

There's a dark side to being a Homeopathist in practice. That is, some consider us to be 'outside the law,' unstructured, anything goes, New Age, so to speak. In fact, Homeopathy is Western - German in origin, refined, challenging, rigorous, intrinsically law abiding. In England, we have a Royal Charter – by reason of the Homeopathic cure of haemophilia in Queen Victoria's grandchild.

All the Royals, to my knowledge, enjoy robust health now, courtesy of Britain's fine Homeopathists. The contrast between the presence of haemophilia on the German Hanovers' family tree and that of their British cousins is one of the best affirmations possible of Homeopathy's profound genetic impact.

To those who take the time to really study it, and understand Hahnemann's inspiration, its impact is so awesome that one wonders if a 'Divine hand' is protecting it from 'profane' users.

The average life span on the Homeopathic practitioner is 85 years, according to Dr. Marjorie Blackie, late Homeopathist to HRH Queen Elizabeth, noting that many of said practitioners find Homeopathy after orthodoxy fails to effect positive change in their own chronic ill health.

The average life span of the orthodox allopath, is 65 years. That may be extended in recent decades, since they have adopted so much of our lateral health enhancement recommendations.

Taking the bathwater, but ignoring the 'baby!'

The Cinchona bark which provided the 'Eureka' moment for Samuel Hahnemann, apothecary and doctor, came from Peru. It was named for the Countess of Cinchon, a benefactor of Surgeon and Saint Martin de Porres beloved poor. St. Martin gave it to Jesuit missionaries who gave brought it to Rome, thence Germany, where became known as *quinine.*

Baffled by a friend's prolonged quotidian (daily) fevers, and prolonged ill health, Hahnemann noted that the symptoms expressed by his friend corresponded to symptoms caused by the over use of quinine. His, friend, however, had not used quinine. Hippocrates, Galen, Pliny, often speculated on what Hahnemann later termed the Law of Similars, ie, 'that which causes, cures,' or 'Like cures Like' and administered quinine to his friend, with spectacular results.

He then closed his practice and gathered the finest physicians in Leipzig to embark on the most intense investigation of the properties of plant, animal and mineral life *ever* to take place on this planet.

This was not publicly funded. Nor was it a private, profit embarking enterprise. It was pure dedication to the service of human kind.

Needless to say, human kind has not yet paid Hahnemann his dues, even refusing to acknowledge the *explosion* that took place within orthodoxy in response to Hahnemann's published findings.

Jenner, Pasteur, Semmelweiss, Freud, and other notables, took inspiration from his work, but picked and poked, and sometimes, distorted his discoveries.

Fortunately for the world, top Ivy League graduates got together, formed the first professional medical body in the United States, and formed The Society of Homeopaths.

This was followed a few years later, by the American Medical Association, or AMA, funded by Big Pharma with the sole intent of suppressing Homeopathy.

If it is from God, it will prevail. Gamaliel principle.

It's from God.

It prevails.

That we practice 'on the fringes' sometimes, is more reflective of the greed and lawlessness of a Pharmaceutical Industry that prioritises profit over patient, and spends a fortune to demean other, time proven healing systems – *at the expense of humanity, even while recalling their own products time and again.*

So much for the highly vaunted 'double blind test,' which cannot be applied to Homeopathy, any more than it can to acupuncture.

In some ways, however, our seemingly marginalised status can put us in a position of discovery, as shadowy figures appear in our waiting rooms, or at the other end of a phone line.

Or it can lead to a request for help by a Head of State.

Above all the pros and cons is the joy of seeing a patient restored to health, without pain, intrusive protocols, side effects, etc., - especially an infant or child.

From time to time I would volunteer with a youth group in the predominantly Hispanic South Bronx. There I encountered a young man, seemingly steeped in prayer and piety, whom I had seen at other youth assemblies.

He asked if he could come to me for counselling, said he didn't have the means to pay.

Although he had wealthy benefactors who offered him scholarships and paid for his transportation to various events, I agreed to treat him *pro bono.* He had some physical problems where I hoped to put Homeopathy to good use.

He survived a sad and tragic childhood. Signed his soul away to the occult. Said he had reclaimed it and converted his life.

That was the first session.

When he arrived for the second session, he was challenging, combative. I could work with that and through that.

I could not work with his triumphalist declaration that he attended the youth events and conferences to gain access to young Hispanic boys as he marched out the door for the last time.

The youth group was so advised. For the safety of the children, first, then for his own safety. If the older brothers learned of his intent, the pietistic pedophile would be floating down the East River minus a body part or three.

Mandated reporting is the law. Sometimes the law is, as Mr. Micawber (Dickens character) says, an 'ass.'

Sometimes it can inhibit a search for guidance or clarification. Sometimes it makes sense and saves lives.

Here, I hope it had the intended result, but with his slew of well to do patrons and clerical psychologist friends to defend him and vilify the 'New Age' Homeopath, he may still be on the loose.

We 'does our best,' so to speak, and when a distinguished Ivy League friend and Cardio Pulmonary Surgeon continued to limp months after a sprain on the ski slopes I offered to help.

With a giant dose of scepticism he accepted my assistance – as a challenge and with a bet against his own recovery.

Needless to say, I won the bet, but instead of being happy he was peeved to the hilt!

An honourable man, however, he coughed up and while we've lost touch, I believe we are still friends!

And, as far as I know, he is still skiing!

As Oscar Wilde once put it – 'There are no grateful people, only resentful ones!'

Sad for Oscar. I know mostly appreciative, loving patients, whom I see as Gift and for whom I am eternally grateful.

Going 'off piste' where rules are concerned, I made some recommendations for the close friend of dear friend and advocate of Homeopathy, a woman whom I admire greatly.

This friend was a biologist who suffered from severe sinusitis and a variety of plant allergies.

His condition improved considerably.

Of course, being a biologist he wanted to know who, what and why.

As many well-meaning people believe that Homeopathy is something found in 'Grandmother's kitchen,' there's a cognitive dissonance of cosmic proportions between popular impressions and the experts' opinion that it 'takes 10 years to make a Homeopathist.'

He was baffled because the remedy used was indeed 'something found in Grandmother's kitchen.'

However, it had been micro diluted, succussed or 'dynamised' at every step and stage, 'proven,' then 'proven' again.

It could then create an 'echo' of the effects caused by over use of the material version, and also cure all 'similar' effects.

Years ago, when Homeopathic remedies were all but impossible to obtain in NYC, the usher at St. Patrick's Cathedral walked me and my young son to the front row, just as Cardinal O'Connor ascended the pulpit to preach the Easter Sunday Homily.

And just as my young son started to sneeze and sneeze and sneeze, in complete harmony with the late, great, Cardinal O'Connor, who did not, however, bat an eye.

No withering glances from *his* pulpit! I knew him as one of the kindest, most patient and tolerant men on the planet.

The front row was decorated with a huge bank of *Azaleas,* but we were blocked and could not leave.

He also suffered from hay fever and cat allergies, so when I returned home, I took samples of all the plants in my courtyard, pollen if possible, leaf where not, and along with an azalea petal from the Cathedral, crushed, diluted, succussed them all until I had a 3x dilution, and administered a few drops.

For the next three summers, no allergies. By that time, Commercial Homeopathic preparations became available in New York.

As an adult he can walk in the woods with impunity and has three cats, no allergies!

The late, great, Cardinal O'Connor opened the door to Homeopathy at a Catholic Hospital.

He arranged a meeting between the female Director of Health and Hospital Services, whom I found cold and hostile and her cohort; myself, Dr. John Vecchione and the son of a European Homeopathic Pharmaceutical Company.

The Cardinal was not present at this meeting.

As cold as the Director was, I was not prepared for the blatant sabotage of the heir apparent of said Pharmaceutical.

He was the first in his family line to study Business rather than Pharmacy, so even if his heart wasn't in Homeopathy, he should have recognised the incredible opportunity when it presented itself to him.

MARY HAD A LITTLE DOG – OR THE END AT THE BEGINNING

My first patient after I re-opened my practice in New York was a remarkable woman.

While she was a registered patient, I would like to pay tribute to her, without violating her confidence. This is not about her condition or health status.

She had the voice of an opera singer, a powerful, natural mezzo soprano, and the heart of an angel.

She loved babies, children, life and 'creatures great and small' and dedicated her life to the care and protection of the vulnerable.

She asked if I could help her dog with his sight, but that was beyond my ability at that point.

She refused to have the little dog put down but knew he only had a few months to live.

Winter was imminent, and the New York ground would be frozen. She was not about to throw the body of her lifelong companion into the trash, preferring to see his final place of rest where he once chased squirrels and where she could visit after his passing.

The care she took of the little fellow was heart-rending and exemplary; so many children, spouses, patients, could use that level of care and attention. Indeed, the world would be a far far better place if my friend Mary's heart was 'the norm.'

It isn't.

We devised a strategy whereby Mary and her friend would go into the park at night, with a flashlight, dig a little by his favourite tree, stuff plastic bags in the cavity, and cover it with a sheet of ply-wood, grass and twigs – easier to remove than frozen mud.

After a couple of nights, the tiny grave was ready. They were not disturbed by any patrols or busy bodies.

Mary returned to her tender care of the little dog, and one icy December morning, called to say that her faithful companion had died, and that she and friend had buried him under his favourite tree, and that all had gone as planned.

She took the loss well, being a person of Faith, and soon her apartment was filled with other happy animals, rescued from shelters and lonely, unloved death by injection.

Her example is humbling.

Ad multos annos, Mary!

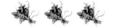

Remedies used in the vignettes:

Arnica Montana

Arsenicum Album

Bryonia

Causticum

Cocculus

Histaminum

Natrum Muriaticum

Nux Vomica

Rhus Toxicondren

Ruta Graveolens

Homeopathy was developed in the late eighteenth century by Dr. Samuel Hahnemann of Leipzig.

He was qualified as both physician and pharmacist.

The great Greek physicians, Hippocrates, Pliny, Galen, all pondered the principle of 'Like curing Like,' ie, symptoms caused by herbs that were also used to cure similar symptoms when unprovoked by said herb.

When his friend fell ill with quotidian fever, he observed that his symptoms were similar to those of quinine poisoning.

Quinine used to be called Cinchona. Cinchona bark was discovered by Surgeon-Friar St. Martin de Porres who named it after the Countess of Cinchon, a benefactor of his beloved poor.

He sent it to Europe via Jesuit Missionaries where two centuries later it became the foundation for the most thoroughly researched, most profound and most effective form of healing the world has ever seen, the dynamic therapies of HOMEOPATHY!

The publication of his pivotal work, 'The Organon' was met with awe, fear, fascination, respect, and horror by arrogant profiteers preying on the sick. It inspired an explosive response – giving orthodox medicine new fields of study – immunology, nutrition, genetics, psychosomatics, and new, kinder treatments for the sick and suffering. Like it or not, Jenner, Breuer-Freud, Semmelweiss, Lister, et al all followed Hahnemann – but could not completely cross over.

Many did, however, and in the USA, The Society of Homeopaths was the first professional medical body, attracting top students from the Ivy Leagues. Homeopathy was used effectively in the Civil War, and in the 1918 global 'flu' epidemic – a 'flu' developing from the poverty, horror, deprivation, malnutrition, stress, lack of shelter, destruction, fear that followed WWI and the Bolshevik Revolution. Homeopathy's patients had a remarkably higher survival rate than orthodoxy despite allegedly getting patients dumped out of orthodox's hospitals. In recognition of which, Homeopathy's patients received discounts from New York's Insurance Companies! Longer lives, fewer problems!

GOLDWATER MEMORIAL HOSPITAL
NEW YORK CITY HEALTH AND HOSPITALS CORPORATION
FRANKLIN D. ROOSEVELT ISLAND, NEW YORK 10044
TELEPHONE: (212) 750-6800

12/28/93

To whom it may concern:

_____ a patient at Goldwater Memorial Hospital has a diagnosis of Cerebral Thrombosis with left hemiplegia, dysarthria and dysphagia. He has also CAD for with he has had by-pass surgery. He has had multiple problems with urinary tract infections and aspiration pneumonias. His multiple antibiotic regimens have given him funguria + fungemia.

I took the liberty to ask Dr. Deidrea McNamara to see him in consultation. She is a homeopathic practitioner and has been seeing him since October 1993 on a weekly basis.

The patient is now stronger, off his ventilator and afebrile. His urine has remained clear without antibiotics; he has gained weight and is being considered for diaphragmatic stimulation for his central sleep apnea.

Medical Director, Respiratory Care

John Vecchione, M.D.

121

About the Author:
Deirdre McNamara discovered Hahnemann's 'Gift of a Gracious God' -Homeopathy - after a childhood and adolescence of protracted illness.

Homeopathy cured! Homeopathy restored to health!

She embarked on an extensive study and opened a practice in New York City where she became the first Homeopathist in nearabouts a century to consult professionally in a New York Hospital.

She particularly honors Dr. John Vecchione, former Medical Director of Goldwater Memorial Hospital for making his patients' well-being a priority and for inviting her to embark on a research project using Homeopathic protocols to wean patients off respirators.

'The Tuscany Express' – will hopefully show how effective and gentle this intensive therapy can be.

Before primitive science and political corruption closed our hospitals, our mortality rate was lower - despite accepting the patients unwanted by allopathy. We still have the most thoroughly researched Materia Medica and highly dedicated practitioners despite our exclusion from the professional, financial and social supports enjoyed by orthodoxy.

And - according to the late physician to HM Queen Elizabeth, Dr. Marjorie Blackie, MD, Homeopathist, we have the greatest longevity - and a Royal Charter in England.

To your good health!

CPSIA information can be obtained at www.ICGtesting.com
Printed in the USA
LVOW09s2110250816

501862LV00022B/217/P

9 781495 431203